INTERMITTENT FASTING FOR WOMEN OVER 50

The Best Way To Accelerate Weight Loss And Reset Your Metabolism. It Only Takes A Few Hours Without Food To Obtain Immediate Results

Health Line Nutrition

Table of Contents

Introduction

No doubt you've heard of intermittent fasting, but how many of you know what it is? Too many people fixate about the word "fasting" and assume that it means going without food for days on end, ignoring the word "intermittent." While it is about going without food for a period of time, it generally doesn't involve days of starving yourself, unless you want to of course, but that's not a healthy way to lose weight.

Intermittent fasting is all about alternate cycles of eating and fasting and plenty of studies have shown that this really works for weight loss, not to mention all the other health benefits that come with it, but only if you do it right.

So, what, exactly, is intermittent fasting?

It is nothing more than a pattern of eating where you eat and then you fast. Rather than being about what you eat, which is what many diets are based on, it focuses more on when you eat, although you do need to be a bit careful about what goes down your throat!

There are also several methods to choose for, most of which are suitable for women and all of them divide the day or the week down into periods of eating and periods of fasting. If you think about it, you already fast for part of the day when you sleep and intermittent fasting is all about going just that little bit longer without food. The easiest way is to miss breakfast, eat at lunchtime and again by about 8 p.m. - Technically that means you are fasting for around 16 hours every day, eating all your meals in a period of 8 hours, the most popular way of doing intermittent fasting.

You might think it's hard to go without food for so long, but it isn't. In fact, you are likely to find that your energy levels are much higher. But I'll get hungry, I hear you whine, I'll starve to death! No you won't. Yes, to start with, hunger will kick in, but that's only because your body has become used to a never-ending stream of food; eventually though, it will learn to accept this new way of eating and the hunger pangs will disappear.

Not all forms of intermittent fasting ban food. Some will allow you to only drink tea, coffee, water and other drinks with no calories but some will allow small amounts of certain foods, and supplements are allowed too, provided they have no calories, because, as I will explain later, it's all about the caloric deficit.

Why would you want to fast, though? Surely it's an unnatural way of eating?

Actually, as a race, we've been doing it for many thousands of years. Of course, sometimes it was because there simply wasn't any food available, but it was also done in the name of religion. Many religions, such as Buddhism, Islam and Christianity all have some form of fasting.

And you've done it yourself. When you were ill, you probably didn't really feel like eating very much, if at all.

So it's clear that intermittent fasting is far from being unnatural and the human body can cope with it very well. And there are loads of benefits to it as well, which I'll divulge later.

For some people, intermittent fasting is a way of life and it makes things easier all around. You don't have to worry about eating several times a day. You only have to plan one or two meals at most per day and that means less prep and less cleaning! Think of the time you can save!

One very important thing to note is that intermittent fasting works differently for women than it does men and not all women will benefit from it. But, for the most part, it is very successful as a way of losing weight, feeling more energetic and being healthier overall. The reason why some women don't fare well on intermittent fasting is that their bodies are far more sensitive to restrictions in calories.

When calories are restricted too much, i.e., when you fast for too long or you do it too often, the hypothalamus in the brain is affected. This, in turn, has an effect on how much GnRH (gonadotropin-releasing hormone) is secreted. GnRH is responsible for the release of two very important reproductive hormones – FSH (follicle stimulating hormone) and KH (luteinizing hormone). If there is little to no communication between these hormones and the ovaries, it can cause issues like irregular menstrual cycle, bad bones, infertility and many other health issues.

As this book is about intermittent fasting for women though I'll only be telling you about the safe methods and how to do them to avoid most, if not all, of these issues.

Intermittent Fasting

1.1   What is Intermittent Fasting

Let's get right to the point. Fasting is a relatively simple practice that yields incredible and complicated results. The effects that fasting has on the body and mind seem unfathomable: weight loss, blood sugar regulation, blood pressure regulation, and growth hormone regulation – only to name a few important ones. In recent years, science has come full force to support these claims, not to mention the thousands of videos online of people's results now that fasting has hit the mainstream. There are different types of fasting as well as many ways to fast.

Within the abundant array of different methods and individual changes any one person may implement, there is a wealth of potential ways to impact the health of the body and mind in positive ways. Fasting, in a general and broad definition, is the practice of willingly abstaining from something, usually food and drink. Whether it is simply not eating chocolate for a week or two or even cutting out all solid foods for a month, no matter how large or small the impact the abstinence has on you, that is fasting from your chosen food. Another more intensive fast would be dry fasting. Dry fasting is the complete abstinence from every source of solid or liquid food for any predetermined period, and, of course, willingly. Although not completely out of the question for beginners, these styles of fasting are used more sparingly than the style we aim to focus on, and that practice is called Intermittent Fasting or IF for short.

IF is very similar to the practices described above, but instead of completely fasting for days at a time, you would choose a certain time of the day, say an eight-hour period. This time window would be the only time you ingest foods as much as you'd like depending on your personal goals. There may also be other rules you set yourself, but there's more on customizing your practice later in the book. The idea of intentionally choosing not to eat may be contradictory to many of the views on food that our culture holds dear. Abundance and indulgence run rampant in our world, and the more you have, the better, right? Not so much. As we now see the results of the destructive habits we have formed, we must look to other answers, better practices, and mindful analyzation of what and when we eat. Changing our eating habit is no small feat; it takes a strong will and a desire to attain a more meaningful and healthy life, one that is not overburdened with sugary snacks and stress caused by overeating. As we can see, IF is not so much a new fad diet but a distinct and progressive lifestyle choice. And although these practices have only recently hit the mainstream in our world today, there is a long and fruitful lineage of practices from cultures all around the world that practiced fasting, and we look to these cultures and our distant ancestors for inspiration and guidance on this journey.

Before today's fast-paced society took hold of our diets, fasting played a very important role in essentially every culture and society around the world. Whether it was for spiritual purposes, health reasons, or some intense ritual, fasting was a lynchpin in many lifestyles throughout human history. Even before humans had science to explore the details of how our bodies work on a microscopic level, we knew that fasting was a source of good health and wellbeing. Primitive cultures would often require fasting before battles and even as an initiatory milestone during puberty. The prehistorical humans surely weren't as concerned about their weight and appearances as we are now, but the hunter-gatherer lifestyle would seemingly fit nicely within the scope of IF. Wandering place to place in search of nutrients, there may have been plenty of time in between meals, but is this fasting? Sure, the ancient tribes probably went long periods without food but probably not willingly. It's impossible to truly find out what the ancient cultures were thinking and practicing, but here, we see potential caloric restriction that influenced early man in incredible ways, perhaps even influencing the onset of agriculture and settling.

As humans progressed and began settling, we see a more prominent and definitive practice of fasting. We see all the big hitters in the religious world advocating for it; Jesus Christ, Muhammed, and Buddha all viewed fasting as a purification process. Commonly based on religious grounds, fasting became a practice of sacrifice, giving up something to show a respected god or entity that you were devoted and deserved good graces from powerful beings. The idea of giving up something so precious, which was required to survive, would surely appease the gods. Certainly, as these practices caught on, the humans, religious or not, felt the results of their fasts. Fasting stays a prominent aspect of medicine as the timeline progresses onward into some ancient cultures that we have better historical documentation of.

The ancient Greek philosophers valued fasting among their other important contributions to our current world. Hippocrates, the father of modern medicine, focused heavily on fasting for a balanced and healthful life. He spoke and promoted the practice while also prescribing it to his patients. The Greek philosophy drew heavily from nature; the observation that humans lose their appetite when they are sick showed the Greek philosophers and doctors that the body naturally restricts caloric intake when ill, and thus there must be some value to the healing potential of willingly abstaining from caloric intake. Another father of contemporary medicine who advocated for fasting was Paracelsus, the inventor of toxicology. He wrote, "Fasting is the greatest remedy, the physician within." The reference to "the physician within" alludes to the body having a natural ability to intuitively heal itself, let alone have assistance by the human mind through the willingness to abstain and attention to the nuances of the mind-body connection. These ancient ideas helped build the foundation of our current state of medicine, but perhaps we need to return to the ideas held dear to our ancestors.

While considering that our ancient ancestors and some of the most prominent minds of our time utilized IF as a means of attaining optimal health, we look forward to today's world. Although the Western world relies heavily on processed foods and a constant intake of foods throughout the day, many contemporary societies live quite the opposite and thrive just as well or even better. One example that stands out is the Hunzakuts of Northern Pakistan. Thriving in the Hunza valley, these people are well known to live well past one hundred years of age, even documenting one woman who was 130 years old! Along with this incredible longevity, the Hunza are living without hardly any degenerative disease. With their diets being high in mineral content and low in sodium, their longevity can be attributed to this, but there is another key factor that suits our purposes. The Hunza people have a very limited food intake. Even without the complicated science and meal plans, they have withheld a standard of longevity quite naturally. Their recent history before being touched by civilization had very interesting patterns that they adhered to not out of choice but simply because that was how they lived their lives. The Hunza people's annual harvest each year would be exhausted, and they would live with minimal caloric intake for weeks at a time each spring. Once the last year's food supply was depleted, they would have minimal sustenance until the new harvest began. With more modern science showing that limited caloric intake has amazing effects on the body and brain, as we will explore, the longevity of the Hunza is linked to their IF lifestyle, along with their distinct diet.

So, around the world, we see fasting being used for survival and necessity, but what about fasting for other purposes? IF finds itself permeating so many aspects of our culture that it cannot be ignored as a key element in human life and survival.

Today, we see fasting prominent in the most widely practiced religions. These holidays and traditions permeate all of the cultures in our interconnected world. Ramadan is a holy month in Islamic religions, during the ninth month of their calendar adherents fast from dawn to dusk – this is IF at its core. Christianity has its holy fast called Lent. This six-week period begins on Ash Wednesday and ends on Easter Sunday, where during this time, there are many celebrations and practices, but fasting remains a very important aspect. For Jewish cultures, Yom Kippur stands out as an important fast day, comprised of a 25-hour fast and intensive prayer. These examples being the most popular, let's not forget that all religions and cultures use fasting. The non-religious and more fact-based mind benefit from fasting's rigorous power to change and alter health. Mahatma Gandhi famously undertook seventeen fasts while fighting for India's independence, showing that fasting isn't simply for health or religious benefit, but can be used to usher in revolution and political change. However, what about all of us who aren't religious adherents or world-changing revolutionaries?

The history of fasting lays a solid foundation that cannot be ignored in modern times. New science technology is confirming the history and reassuring contemporary populations that IF is a safe, effective, and simple path to overall health. Not only is fasting resting comfortably on the shoulders of science and history, but it also has perks in the consumerist world we live in. Since fasting requires no prescriptions, no fitness contraptions, and no expensive supplements, the practice fits nicely within our money-hungry, materialist society. Simply abstaining from something you love to eat for a day or two changes your outlook on your potential to take control of your life and literally will save you money as you will be consuming less than usual. As practical as it sounds, many feel that it is too good to be true, that simply not eating could not possibly affect the body and brain as much as people claim. And sure, at first glance, it seems like a gimmick that celebrity doctors want to scam you with, but given the test of time and solid science, fasting will remain a pivotal practice in the rearranging of our lives in the Western world, an action that desperately needs to be put into play.

Now that we've gotten acquainted with the history and basics of fasting and its role in our society let's focus on some in-depth science on IF to truly grasp what will happen when we begin this amazing journey of transformation.

1.2   How Intermittent Fasting Works

Intermittent Fasting is interval starvation when only liquid is allowed for 12-24 (36) hours. Many supporters of such a diet have noted the improvement in their own well-being, weight loss, and other health benefits. Many studies have been conducted aimed at identifying these advantages. MedAboutme will tell you about the results. Slimming Intermittent fasting promotes weight loss due to the work of insulin. During its life, the body splits carbohydrates into glucose. It is the main source of energy for cells. To absorb glucose, insulin is needed. It is a hormone that is produced by the pancreas. Insulin concentration decreases during fasting, and just this reduction contributes to the fact that the cells begin to release their accumulated energy to maintain metabolic processes and vital functions. Regular repetition of this process ensures slimming. But you should not expect quick results. But the results are durable. It is noted that the observance of intermittent fasting, in general, leads to the consumption of fewer calories, which also ensures weight loss. The journal Molecular and Cellular Endocrinology for 2015 published an analysis of more than 40 studies on intermittent fasting and its health benefits. Scientists have concluded that the observance of fasting not only contributes to weight loss but also ensures the proper functioning of organs and systems, as well as metabolic processes. In studies conducted in 2017, the effect of intermittent fasting and diet with calorie restriction on weight loss for 12 months was compared. The data showed: fasting and dieting were equally effective.

Numerous studies have shown that adherence to intermittent fasting is an effective weight loss strategy. A significant advantage is a fact that intermittent fasting is much easier to follow than some types of diets. Less often there are no breakdowns, and the result of losing weight is long lasting. Diabetes Prevention Diabetes is a chronically dangerous disease with many complications and health effects. It is known that overweight is one of the risk factors for its development, and compliance with intermittent fasting will contribute to its prevention. In 2014, Translational Research published studies proving that intermittent fasting contributes to a decrease in blood glucose levels. Intermittent fasting is promising in the prevention of type II diabetes, but more research is needed to confirm this data and study cause-effect relationships. The data showed a reduction in the level of markers of diabetes, such as insulin resistance in overweight and obese patients. But there is a reverse point of view: in 2018, Endocrine Abstracts published data from rodent studies that proved that intermittent fasting may increase the risks of diabetes. During the study, it was observed that in rodents there was a decrease in weight and food intake, but at the same time the amount of adipose tissue in the abdominal cavity and the decrease in muscle volume increased; thus, it was possible to identify signs that insulin is not being used properly. These are known risk factors for type II diabetes. Whether the diabetes is threatening with Intermittent Fasting remains to be seen. This issue is addressed by a whole group of scientists from around the world. It is also necessary to find out whether the results obtained in rodents are applicable to humans. Improving heart health Doctors concluded that intermittent fasting contributes to the health of the heart and blood vessels. A review of studies for 2016 reported that intermittent fasting reduces blood pressure, normalizes heart rate, and reduces the concentration of "harmful" cholesterol in the blood. The data were confirmed both in animals and in humans. Brainwork Mice that were on intermittent fasting demonstrated better learning and memory compared to those who had free access to food without restriction. Other studies have shown that intermittent fasting reduces the risks of numerous diseases and neurological conditions, including Alzheimer's disease, Parkinson's, and even stroke. The research results were obtained in the study of rodents, in the future to prove the consistency of this theory in relation to people.

Reducing the risk of cancer pathologies.

Studies were conducted for a long time. And the results of studies on living animals showed that the stingy post can slow down (and even stopping in non-major cases) the occurrence and development of tumors. Everyone is aware of the fact that people who are overweight are at risk for many types of cancer. Therefore, diet can be considered as a factor that reduces the risks of cancer development. In addition, adherence to intermittent fasting can reduce some of the biological factors associated with cancer. But to confirm the data and identify the causal relationship, it is necessary to conduct several additional studies.

1.3   Benefits of Intermittent Fasting

Weight loss is probably the main reason why this diet is quite popular. Weight loss is a great benefit, but this diet offers more than just this. In this section, you will learn about the different benefits of this popular dieting protocol.

Lose Weight

The most popular and obvious benefit of intermittent fasting is weight loss. Intermittent fasting oscillates between eating and fasting periods. This obviously results in a reduction of your total calorie intake. Unless you go overboard and try to compensate for the fasting hours by binging too much when you break the fast. Fasting helps with weight loss as well as maintenance of the weight loss. Fasting is also a great way to prevent from indulging in mindless eating. As mentioned earlier, whenever you eat something, your body immediately converts it into glucose and fat. When you skip a meal or two, then your body starts to burn fats to meet the energy requirements. When your body reaches into its internal fat stores, it leads to weight loss. A significant portion of the fat cells is present in the abdominal region. So, if you want a flat tummy, then this is a great diet.

Better Sleep

One of the major health problems these days is obesity.

In fact, obesity is a marker for various diseases and illnesses. Lack of sleep is a primary cause of obesity. Whenever your body is deprived of the rest it needs, then your internal mechanism of burning fats slows down. Intermittent fasting helps regulate your sleep cycle, and it also makes your body's fat burning mechanism effective and efficient. Good sleep has psychological benefits as well. Your energy levels will stay high when you get a good night's sleep.

Improves the Resistance to Illnesses

Intermittent fasting kickstarts autophagy. Autophagy helps with the regeneration and removal of damaged cells. This is a natural process, and intermittent fasting makes it more efficient. This helps to improve the overall functioning of your cellular components. When this happens, then your body is better equipped to deal with illnesses.

Improves Heart Health

Intermittent fasting helps with weight loss and this, in turn, helps improve the functioning of your cardiovascular system. The buildup of plaque is the leading cause of several cardiovascular diseases. The buildup of plaque is known as atherosclerosis, and in this condition, the thin lining of blood vessels (endothelium) don't function effectively. Obesity is one of the major reasons for the increase in plaque deposits. Stress or inflammation tends to worsen this situation even further. By tackling obesity, it directly helps reduce the risk factors associated with cardiovascular diseases and as a result, improves your heart's health.

Improves your Gut's Health

Are you aware that your gut is home to millions of microorganisms? The symbiotic microorganisms are known as microbiome assist the functioning of the digestive system. Intermittent fasting ensures that these microbiomes are functioning optimally and this, in turn, improves the gut's health and improves in better assimilation and absorption of the food you consume.

Managing Diabetes

Diabetes is quite troublesome by itself. It is a primary aggressor for cardiovascular dysfunction that leads to different health problems like heart attacks and strokes. Your body releases insulin whenever you consume food; however when the level of glucose increases in the bloodstream, and there isn't sufficient insulin to deal with it, it causes diabetes. Diabetes also leads to your body developing resistance to insulin, and this makes it difficult for your body to manage insulin levels. Intermittent fasting helps decrease sensitivity to insulin and this, in turn, helps manage diabetes.

Reduces Inflammation

Your body's natural defense mechanism to deal with any internal problems is inflammation. Inflammation is helpful in moderation, and it helps fight off any foreign bodies; however, if left unchecked, inflammation can be quite troublesome. A high level of inflammation causes metabolic dysfunction and leads to different painful conditions like arthritis, atherosclerosis and other degenerative diseases. Such inflammation is known as chronic inflammation, and it is a rather painful condition. Intermittent fasting helps control chronic inflammation.

Promotes Cellular Repair

Intermittent fasting helps kickstart autophagy. Most of the diseases related to the aging of the brain take a long time to develop since the proteins present in and around the brain cells are misfiled, and they don't function like they are supposed to. Autophagy helps clean up all these malfunctioning proteins and reduces the accumulation of such proteins. For instance, in Alzheimer's, autophagy helps remove amyloid and α-synuclein in Parkinson's. In fact, there is a reason why it is believed that dementia and diabetes go hand in hand with each other—the constantly high levels of blood sugar prevent autophagy from kicking in and this makes it quite difficult for the body to get rid of any damaged or malfunctioning cells.

The Six Types of Intermittent Fasting

There are various methods of intermittent fasting, so there is bound to be a method that suits your lifestyle. Some methods are more intense than others, and it is to be noted that the fasts that yield more radical results are generally the fasts that require more radical dedication. However, even small fasts can boost your metabolism and help you see results. Some methods, like the 5:2 diet, do not require a full fast, but rather a large decrease in the number of calories consumed on fast days. The 16:8 diet simply involves skipping one meal a day. These two methods are generally considered the least daunting and are good ways to introduce your body to fasting. Other methods include the "eat - stop – eat" diet (which involves a 24-hour fast once or twice each week), alternate day fasting, and the warrior diet. Which method you choose depends on various factors like your schedule, special events, responsibilities to feed others, biology, weight loss or muscle gain goals, and workout routine. Whatever needs you have to meet, there is a method of intermittent fasting that can suit your life.

2.1 16/8 Intermittent Fasting Method

The 16:8 diet is another method that may allow you to introduce intermittent fasting into your diet without being overwhelmed. The 16 stands for the sixteen-hour "fast" period, and the 8 stands for the eight-hour "fed" period. The 16:8 method basically involves sacrificing one meal a day, and it's up to you whether that meal is in the morning or evening. When you finish eating for the day, you simply wait 16 hours before beginning to eat the next day. If you sleep a standard eight hours a night that already takes care of half of your sixteen-hour fast period! Let's say you wake up in the morning and have a cup of coffee or tea to start your day. Try to avoid adding sugar or milk, but it's widely accepted that if you consume less than 50 calories during the fasting period, your body will continue to benefit from fasting without entering a fed state. So, you can have your morning beverage, and good on you if you can keep your tea or coffee plain. Then around 1 o'clock p.m., you can eat lunch. You can snack if you want in the afternoon, then eat an evening meal. Because you started eating at 1 o'clock, you should finish eating by 9 o'clock that evening. During this eight-hour fed period, you can consume a full day's worth of calories. It's important to ensure that you are staying hydrated between 9 o'clock and 1 o'clock the following afternoon. Water intake should be increased slightly beyond the normal level to compensate for the fluids that would normally be absorbed by food consumption. Flip this schedule if you are a person who really needs to eat in the morning to be fueled for your day. You can break your fast at 8 a.m. and begin fasting again at 4 p.m. This can allow a breakfast, some snacks, and a late lunch, or even a small lunch and an early dinner before you begin fasting again.

Allowing sixteen hours without feeding your body will give it an opportunity to use the calories in the food it has consumed as well as burning stored fat for fuel. You can modify the 16:8 diet to fit into your schedule and meet your personal needs. Many people find this diet to be the least restrictive form of intermittent fasting because it does not require any alteration in the number of calories consumed and a standard meal schedule is able to fit well into an 8-hour block.

2.2 The 5/2 Method of Intermittent Fasting

If completely depriving your body of calories seems too scary, give the 5:2 diet a try. The premise is simple, eat normally for five days out of the week and drastically reduce calorie intake on the remaining two days. For men, it is recommended to consume around 600 calories on fasting days. For women, it is recommended to consume around 500 calories. You can meet this calorie goal with whatever foods you like, but it's recommended to eat vegetables and low-calorie proteins to ensure you are still getting the nutrients your body needs. On the five feeding days, you are allowed to continue on a normal diet. If you are wanting to see quicker results, it's not best to overeat during these five days or to eat foods that will not fuel your body well. Not only can this prevent your body from reaching the caloric deficit you are aiming for, but it also means that on the fasting days, but your body also will not react as well to the reduction in energy. It's also ideal to make sure the fasting days are not consecutive. Eating for five days, then only allowing yourself a total of 1000-1200 calories in the remaining 48 hours can leave the body feeling weak. Separate the two fasting days by making sure there is at least one, if not more, feed day between them. When you are new to fasting, it's not encouraged to jump right in with both feet. Test the waters first by implementing a 5:2 diet. Begin by incorporating one calorie restricted day per week, then work your way up to incorporating two days. If you want to give the 5:2 diet a try but do not know how to get started, worry not. This book contains a 14 day 5:2 diet meal plan that you can follow to begin implementing a 5:2 eating schedule.

Every diet has a few downsides, and some people will struggle more than others. The fact that the 5:2 diet does not require a full fast from calories can actually make it a bit harder to get used to. Meeting a small calorie count rather than avoiding food altogether can leave one feeling hungrier and more focused on the lack of food. Fasting from food in its entirety affects the production of hunger hormones, and over time your body will start to get less hungry during your fasting periods. When you are restricting calories dramatically but still eating, this change in hormones does not occur. You may be left feeling the effects of your hunger much more than someone who chooses another fasting routine. During other methods of fasting, it can also help to distract yourself from the food you are not eating. The 5:2 diet does not allow this quite as much. In fact, if you are serious about your weight loss goals and desire to make the most of your minuscule calorie allotment for the day, you may find that you are even more focused on food than normal. It's also important to note that your fast days should be scheduled on days when you won't be over-exerting yourself. Because you are giving yourself less fuel, intense workouts or high levels of physical exertion will be difficult on the body. Yoga and light exercise like walking may be ideal for the two days during which your calorie count is low.

2.3 Eat-Stop-Eat

If you do not want to fast quite as consistently, try incorporating a 24-hour fast into your diet once or twice a week. This method is called the "eat - stop - eat" diet. The 24 hour fasting period should be scheduled so that you are consuming some form of sustenance every day. For instance, let's say you eat breakfast at 8:30 in the morning on Tuesday morning. You finish eating by 9 o'clock and begin your fast. At 9 o'clock in the morning on Wednesday morning, you can break your fast. Incorporating this type of fasting into your lifestyle once or twice a week can allow the same type of caloric deficit as other methods while not interfering as much with normal day-to-day activities. This method may be ideal if you like to do heavy workouts on many days of the week.

Incorporating fasting on your rest days can allow you to fuel yourself well on work days and decrease consumption on days when you are burning fewer calories. In the same form as other methods, sticking to healthier foods on feast days can help to achieve the results while also avoiding feelings of weakness and lethargy during the fasting period.

The eat - stop - eat method will be helpful in reaching a caloric deficit and losing weight. However, this method may not yield the same caliber of results as others because the fasting is less consistent. The body will remain more accustomed to being in a fed state and therefore not gain quite the same level of benefits as more frequent fasting. It is still an effective method and will still be beneficial to the body's processes. Eat - stop - eat may be a good option for you if you are new to fasting or if you find it difficult to add a fasting schedule into your busy life.

Some people extend their fast little by little until it lasts for a duration of multiple days to increase the amount of time the body is in a fat burning state. Long-term fasting has been shown to dramatically increase levels of the human growth hormone and noradrenaline. These two hormones are essential to fat burning, muscle growth, muscle preservation, energy levels, mental clarity, cellular repair, and anti-aging. Extended fasting also allows the body to enter and remain in a state of ketosis which will burn more stored fat and increase the rapidity of weight loss. It is wise to consult a doctor before incorporating long fasting periods into your lifestyle. For women, fasting for more than 24 hours at a time can have adverse effects on hormone levels and may cause permanent damage to the body. It may also not be smart if you have health problems that affect your blood sugar levels, such as diabetes. This can increase the risk of diabetic ketoacidosis and other potentially harmful illnesses associated with drastic changes in blood glucose levels. When you break your fast, the drastic change in blood sugar can be dangerous. Being aware of what is happening inside of your body is key to approaching fasting healthily. Long-term fasting can be beneficial, but it should not be attempted if your body is not healthy enough for it.

2.4 Alternate - Day Fasting

Alternate day fasting, or the "every other day diet," is fairly self-explanatory. Eat for one full day, fast for one full day, repeat. This does not mean to fast from the moment you wake up until the end of the day but eat three square meals the next day. When practicing alternate day fasting, you should eat at least one meal every day. This may mean eating breakfast before 9 o'clock in the morning then abstaining from food until the same time the next day, or it could involve eating dinner by 7 o'clock in the evening and abstaining until 7 o'clock the following evening. Whatever time works best for you can be the beginning or ending time of your 24-hour fasting and feeding windows. This diet drastically reduces the calorie intake over the whole week because you are removing multiple days' worth of calories from the equation. Fasting for a full day between feast days allows the body to spend more time in a fat burning unfed state. On feasting days, you can eat whatever you'd like. For optimal weight loss, sticking to a healthy diet and not bingeing with carbs or unhealthy snacks is ideal. Some people practice this method with the same caloric restrictions as the 5:2 diet, so on fasting days, they are allowed 500 to 600 calories. Some studies have shown that this level of calorie intake is easier to maintain than full fasts and overall it is similar in effectiveness.

The "every other day" method has not proven to be any more effective than utilizing a diet that involves daily calorie restriction, but some people find it easier to restrict every other day so they can still enjoy an unrestricted diet half of the time. Both will yield similar fat loss results, but the intermittent fasting method has shown more successful in preserving muscle mass. This muscle mass is crucial to the burning of calories. It has also been shown that, in some cases, following this method can cause the body to feel less hungry during restricted periods than it would on a standard, calorie restrictive diet and can decrease the likelihood of binge eating on feast days. Hormones such as ghrelin that cause the body to feel hungry when it is fasting can decrease, and the hormones that cause it to feel satiated increases. The concern with this diet is that intermittent fasting is not always a permanent lifestyle choice and a diet like this can increase the likelihood of bingeing later on. When you are used to a full binge one day and a full restriction the next, you can lose touch with what true hunger or satiety feels like. When you resume consuming food on a daily basis, the eating habits you may have become accustomed to bingeing and may lead to weight gain.

This method is also not ideal for women. The female body reacts differently than the male body to extended periods of fasting. A full 24 hours of fasting is riskier for women, but still within the allowed time frame. Extended fasts in women can change hormone levels drastically and over time can cause permanent damage to the reproductive system, possibly even leading to infertility. If you are a woman who would like to utilize this type of eating schedule, it is possible, but it's important to understand the risks associated with it. It is also important to avoid implementing such a long period of food avoidance if your body is not already accustomed to fasting. Start by fasting for 12 hours, then gradually increase the fasting window until you reach 24 hours to avoid a major shock to the body that can cause hormonal imbalances with potentially dangerous side effects.

2.5 Warrior Diet

One of the more extreme methods of intermittent fasting is the Warrior Diet. The Warrior Diet is based on a theory that humans are biologically built to consume and process food in line with their circadian clock. The diet consists of eating one calorically dense meal every evening and fasting for the rest of the day. This is based around the belief that "warriors" of antiquity spent their time fighting, hunting and generally taking care of business throughout the majority of the day, so they ate much less during that time. Therefore, they would end their days indulging in a larger meal. In this same way, individuals who practice the Warrior Diet fast for the majority of every day. Generally, this follows a 20:4 method, with a twenty-hour fasting window and a four-hour feasting window. During the 4 hours, individuals consume a high number of calories. This can lead some people to choose unhealthy foods, but it is recommended to eat a healthy, balanced meal, especially if you will be exercising during your fasting period. Fueling your body properly will help you get optimal results and stay as healthy as possible while practicing intermittent fasting. During the 20-hour fast period, you do not have to avoid food entirely. Small snacks made up of raw vegetables or fruits, boiled eggs, and dairy products are encouraged, and you can drink as many calorie-free beverages as your warrior's heart desires. This includes tea, coffee, diet sodas, and of course lots and lots of water.

The Warrior Diet was created by an ex-member of the Israeli Special Forces who found inspiration in his time as a soldier and carried his knowledge and experience into the field of fitness and nutrition. However, the creator of this diet admits that it is not based on science and the amount of research around it is nearly non-existent. This does not necessarily mean that it isn't effective, but it is a good point to remember when considering this method.

Many people who practice the Warrior Diet incorporate exercise into their routine during the fasting period. This can be an effective way to build muscle, but it carries potentially harmful side effects. Pushing the body to its limits when it is low on fuel (food) can cause fatigue and dehydration, as well as decreasing your overall ability to perform which may lead to injury. This can also lead to a condition called hypoglycemia which is essentially dangerously low blood sugar. Hypoglycemia can lead to problems of varying severities ranging from confusion, increased clumsiness, trouble forming words, and dizziness to seizures and possible death. If you have type 1 diabetes or are on medication designed to lower your blood sugar, you should never attempt this diet. Again, it is important to consult your doctor before trying to incorporate a fasting regime into your lifestyle. An extended fast such as this also increases the likelihood of binge eating and consuming foods that are not rich in the nutrients necessary to fuel the body. When you are consuming a full day's worth of calories in 4 hours, opting for a carb-heavy meal full of processed food may seem appealing. Ensuring that your body is receiving the proper vitamins and minerals to maintain its functions is crucial to a healthy practice of intermittent fasting. Incorporating a meal prep plan into your Warrior Diet can help to avoid this issue and increase your likelihood of success.

Practicing any method of intermittent fasting is not recommended for people who may suffer from eating disorders. Any restrictive diet is not suggested for people with a tendency to over-restrict calories. Also, most people do not use intermittent fasting as a lifelong commitment, so someday they will probably stop practicing it. After you become accustomed to fasting, eating on a normal schedule can cause unwanted weight gain. You may lose touch with your ability to sense when you are truly hungry or full, and you may become accustomed to eating higher calorie meals. If you are not careful, this may lead to overeating which can bring about feelings of shame or regret that can negatively affect mental health. In individuals who are at risk of disordered eating, the negative emotions connected to this can lead to bingeing and purging behaviors.

Depending on the state of your health, your lifestyle, your weight loss or muscle gain goals, and your reaction to fasting, there is likely a method of intermittent fasting that suits your needs. The 5:2 diet and time restricted eating methods like the 16:8 are ideal for beginners and have much fewer risks attached. If you want fast, drastic results, the Warrior Diet may be ideal for you. All of these methods will help you lose fat. Some will help you lose more fat, more quickly, and some will help you build and maintain muscle mass more effectively. You do not have to stick to one method forever. The beauty of fasting is that it can be done in whatever way suits your lifestyle the best and can be catered individually to your wants and desires.

2.6 Spontaneous Meal Skipping

If you are a beginner wishing to implement this method, you can start by incorporating a larger eating window and gradually shortening it over time. The 16:8 method is part of a group of fasting schedules referred to as "time-restricted eating" which also includes the 12:12 method and 14:10 method. The 12:12 method is very similar to a schedule many people already follow and may be a good start if you've never tried time-restricted eating before. Start with a 12-hour eating window, then after a week, you can take away 2 hours. Now you are practicing the 14:10 method. After another week, give 16:8 a try. Some people even choose to go further with their time restrictions and incorporate an 18:6 or 20:4 schedule.

It is up to you to choose how far you would like to take your schedule restrictions. The most important thing to take into account when considering your options is the health of your body. Take your time in adjusting to fasting to avoid unnecessary stress on the body and always be sure your body is healthy enough for fasting before implementing any changes.

It is important to note that if you wish to incorporate physically demanding exercise into your day, you should be aware of how your body reacts to working out in a fasted state versus a fed state and schedule your meals and workouts accordingly. Some people choose to do fasted workouts for a variety of reasons, and some find that their bodies are simply not adequately fueled for such workouts during the fasting period. Your fasting method should be adapted to suit your life, so pay attention to your body and take it into consideration. Pushing your body to work out when you have less energy due to fasting can lead to ineffective workouts and even injury. Many sports nutritionists advise choosing a fasting schedule that coincides with your ideal workout schedule so you can fuel your body immediately before or after exercise. If you are practicing the 16:8 method by skipping breakfast, this may mean working out in the afternoon or evening. Many people prefer to work out in the morning when human growth hormone levels are naturally highest. If this is the case for you, you may choose to implement your feeding window in the morning and begin your fast in the afternoon rather than the evening.

Foods to Eat & Avoid in Intermittent Fasting

Because you'll likely want to keep your reproductive and menstrual systems working to their best capacities while you engage in intermittent fasting, you'll have to make sure your dietary choices reflect the health you want to see. You won't really want to "diet" all that much, as mentioned above, but you can make certain healthful changes that allow your body to function at its highest capacity *while* it adjusts to intermittent fasting, sheds that excess weight, and reaches a new and purer energy level than you've ever experienced before.

In this chapter, you will be introduced to concepts and details that will help you eat and drink the things that are best suited to your overall growth and success with intermittent fasting. You'll be shown the pros and cons of the intermittent fasting lifestyle, and you'll be taught tips on how to manage hunger and generally achieve your IF goals.

By the end of this section, you should know the best and worst that intermittent fasting has to offer, and you should feel confident that the foods you'll seek during your break from fast will be as health-conscious and supportive as possible, based on the information you've gained. Finally, you should also feel prepared to deal with those "worsts" that IF has to offer through the tips at the end of the chapter. If you're not ready to try intermittent fasting by the end of this section, I'll be incredibly surprised.

Pros & Cons of IF as a Dietary/Lifestyle Choice

On the most basic level (without being too redundant), the pros of switching to intermittent fasting (whether as a lifestyle choice or as more of a simple two-month fasting experiment) include:

- Increased health overall
- through weight loss, lowered insulin & blood sugar levels, heart health, better muscle mass preservation, increased neuroplasticity, potential for cancer healing, lower blood pressure & cholesterol, healthier hormone production, longer life, re-started/re-inspired nutrient absorption, reduced inflammation
- Increased energy, improved mental processing and better access to memory
- Increased overall sense of well-being
- both mentally and as a side-effect of having the body type you want through weight loss
- Eased & regulated menstruation
- including lessened period cramps and potential for lessened fertility
- The ability to retain your current diet and caloric intake
- The overall simplicity and ease of starting and maintaining your IF approach, and the versatility and flexibility of IF as a practice

On the flip-side, the cons associated with intermittent fasting
(as both a lifestyle and momentary dietary choice) include:

- Potential for increased headaches

- These are often caused by dehydration and salt withdrawal from eating less than normal.

- Increase your water intake & mix in a quarter-teaspoon of salt with each water glass, and you'll feel right as rain in no time.

- Potential for constipation

- Just increase your fiber intake to help with this issue!

- Potential for dizziness when in a fasting period

- Look to the final section of this chapter for help in this case.

- Potential for muscle cramps

- Take supplemental magnesium or sit for a while in an Epsom salt bath to cure these "growing" pains.

- Potential for worst-case-scenario side-effects

- This potential is only a concern if IF is not practiced the right way for you and your body.

- potential side-effects include: irregular or ceased menses, hair loss, dry skin/acne, slow healing to injuries, mood swings, super-slow metabolism, constant cold feelings, insomnia, etc.

- Potential to binge when you do eat

- Be conscious of your body and what it can handle!

- Interference with social eating patterns

- It might feel awkward not to eat with everyone else, or to have to explain yourself every time you don't.

- Low energy or unproductivity during fast periods

- This issue can be helped with practice and by eating the right types of foods when you do eat.

- The fact that some of the lasting effects of IF are still largely unstudied or uncertain

- such as: its effects on the heart, on fertility, on breastfeeding women, on stress, etc.

What Foods & Liquids Do

When you go about your first round of intermittent fasting, you'll need to know what to avoid and what to keep close at hand. The following portion of this chapter will reveal exactly what's safe, what to avoid, and what does what for you.

When it comes to foods, the best things to have around are:

- All Legumes and Beans – good carbs can help lower body weight without planned calorie restriction

- Anything high in protein – helpful in keeping your energy levels up in your efforts as a whole, even when you're in a period of fasting

- Anything with the herbs cayenne pepper, psyllium, or dried/crushed dandelion – they'll contribute to weight loss without sacrificing calories or effort

- Avocado – a high-, good-calorie fruit that has a lot of healthy fats

- Berries – often high in antioxidants and vitamin C as well as flavonoids for weight loss

- Cruciferous Vegetables – broccoli, cauliflower, brussel sprouts, and more are incredibly high in fiber, which you'll definitely want to keep constipation at bay with IF

- Eggs – high in protein and great for building muscle during IF periods

- Nuts & Grains – sources of healthy fats and essential fiber

- Potatoes – when prepared in healthy ways, they satiate hunger well and help with weight loss

- Wild-Caught Fish – high in healthy fats while providing protein and vitamin D for your brain

When it comes to liquids, some of it is pretty self-explanatory:

- Water:

- It's always good for you! It will help keep you hydrated, it will provide relief with headaches or lightheadedness or fatigue, and it clears out your system in the initial detox period.

- Try adding a squeeze of lemon, some cucumber or strawberry slices, or a couple of sprigs of mint, lavender, or basil to give your water some flavor if you're not enthused with the taste of it plain.

- If you need something other than water to drink, you can always seek out:

- Probiotic drinks like kefir or kombucha

- You can even look for probiotic foods such as sauerkraut, kimchi, miso, pickles, yogurt, tempeh, and more!

- Probiotics work amazingly well at healing your gut especially in times of intense transition, as with the start of intermittent fasting.

- Black coffee

- Sweeteners and milk aren't productive for your

fasting and weight loss goals.

- Try black coffee whenever possible, in moderation.
- Heated or chilled vegetable or bone broths
- Teas of any kind
- Apple cider vinegar shots
- Instead, try water or other drinks with ACV mixed in.

Drinks to avoid would be:

- Regular soda
- Diet soda
- Alcohol of any kind
- High-sugar coconut and almond drinks
- i.e. coconut water, coconut milk, almond milk, etc.
- Go for the low-sugar or unsweetened milk alternative if it's available.
- Anything with artificial sweetener
- Artificial sweetener will shock your insulin levels into imbalance with your blood sugar later on.

Managing Hunger & Other Useful Tips

A few supportive tips to help troubleshoot, keep inspired and stay focused as you may happen to encounter the "cons" of intermittent fasting are as follows.

Generally, keep these pointers in mind: don't over-exercise and over-limit yourself with calorie intake or with food when you do breakfast. Take pictures of your progress to help keep the inspiration flowing, try not to binge when you breakfast and make sure to do your proper research or check with your doctor to be sure your plan for intermittent fasting is really the right one for you!

When it comes to managing hunger, the best thing to do is think of hunger like a wave passing over you. Sometimes the build-up to that wave seems unbearable, but it will crest and crash eventually, passing completely over and through you. If you wait it out, keep yourself busy, and take a few sips of a drink instead. You'll find that these hunger pangs are bearable and not quite as overwhelming as they were at the start. By the end of the third day, you should have a significantly increased capacity to handle these feelings of hunger.

If you start feeling dizzy or lightheaded, one of two things is likely happening to you. You may be experiencing low blood volume, or you might be experiencing low blood *pressure* instead. Just drinking water, in this case, might not help you all that much; in fact, if you just drink water, you'll be diluting the number of electrolytes in your system even more, so try mixing a bit of sea salt in your water instead. Frequently, for those who don't experience dizziness or lightheadedness unless they're intermittently fasting, this addition of sea salt to water does the trick. However, some people were liable to feel dizzy or lightheaded before they ever tried IF. For those people (or for those for whom mixing salt into their water doesn't help), taking magnesium supplements can also work well, and if that still doesn't help, the issue could be something else entirely. Possible adrenal weakness, anemia, or low blood sugar would most likely be the cause in this case.

If your period gets lighter or starts to disappear, make sure you're getting enough fat in your diet when you fast! If you **had** been limiting calorie intake, stop doing that right now, and be sure not to binge (on the opposite extreme). Just eat what you would if you weren't IF or dieting at all. These slight adjustments should help resolve this issue. If not, seek advice from your doctor.

When you notice you've become moodier, there are a couple of things you can do to help and troubleshoot the issue. First things first, don't open yourself up to negative moods by keeping the information about your eating pattern shift to yourself and people you really trust. Some people will bombard you with questions, hate, or confusion when you tell them about your work with IF, and you should remember that you **don't** have to tell anyone who you think won't support you.

Second, you can make sure you're not still in the detox period of intermittent fasting! During the first few weeks, you'll be working through the detox period that brings up lots of literal stink and emotional issues to boot. Bear through the trial period and see if that moodiness lingers. If you're still frustratingly and unusually moody after week two is complete, you might just have low blood sugar. Work to counteract low blood sugar through the foods you choose to eat when you breakfast, and the issue should clear itself up in no time.

Finally, two pieces of advice are left, and they're some of the most important ones to internalize. First, **choose a plan that starts small and incorporates your life in its planning**! If you sleep for almost 12 hours each night anyway, the 16:8 method might be best for you. If you wake early without much sleep constantly, you might be better off doing alternate-day fasting. Go with what works for your schedule, and things will start off so much smoother than they would otherwise.

Second and lastly, **start with one month and be open; see what happens**! You're bound to get frustrated and moody after and during the first week but commit to withstand the awkwardness and at least get through the first two weeks to the beginning of week three. Stick with it and wait to see what this unintentional cleanse has in store for you.

Intermittent Fasting Appetizer & Snack Recipes

Chicken Popcorns

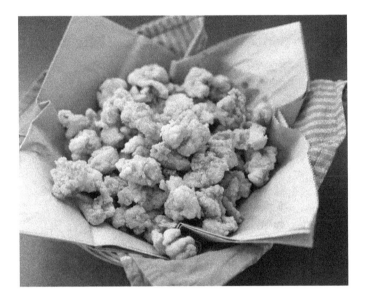

Total time: 40 minutes

Ingredients:

½ pound grass-fed chicken thigh, cut into bite-sized pieces

7 ounces unsweetened coconut milk

1 teaspoon ground turmeric

Salt and ground black pepper, as required

2 tablespoons coconut flour

3 tablespoons desiccated coconut

1 tablespoon coconut oil, melted

Directions

Place the chicken, coconut milk, turmeric, salt and black pepper in a large bowl and mix well.

Cover the bowl and refrigerate to marinate overnight.

Preheat the oven to 390 degrees F.

Place the coconut flour and desiccated coconut in a shallow dish and mix well.

Coat the chicken pieces evenly with coconut mixture.

Arrange the chicken piece onto a baking sheet and drizzle with oil.

Bake for about 20-25 minutes.

Remove the baking sheet from oven and transfer the chicken popcorn onto a platter.

Set aside to cool slightly.

Serve warm.

Chicken Nuggets

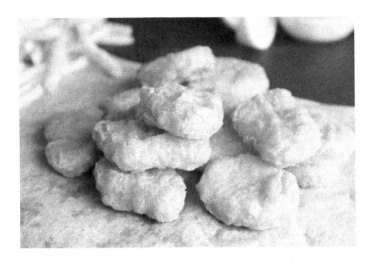

Total time: 45 minutes

Ingredients:

2 (8-ounces) grass-fed skinless, boneless chicken breasts, cut into 2x1-inch chunks

2 organic eggs

1 cup almond flour

1 teaspoon dried oregano, crushed

½ teaspoon onion powder

½ teaspoon garlic powder

½ teaspoon paprika

Salt and ground black pepper, as required

Directions

Preheat the oven to 350 degrees F. Grease a baking sheet.

Crack the eggs in a shallow bowl and beat well.

Place the flour, oregano, spices, salt, and black pepper in another shallow bowl and mix until well combined.

Dip the chicken nuggets in beaten eggs and then, evenly coat with the flour mixture.

Arrange the chicken nuggets onto prepared baking sheet in a single layer.

Bake for about 30 minutes or until golden brown.

Remove from the oven and set aside to cool slightly.

Serve warm.

Tuna Croquettes

Total time: 31 minutes

Ingredients:

24 ounces canned white tuna, drained

¼ cup mayonnaise

4 large organic eggs

2 tablespoons yellow onion, finely chopped

1 scallion, thinly sliced

4 garlic cloves, minced

¾ cup almond flour

Salt and ground black pepper, as required

¼ cup olive oil

Directions

Place the tuna, mayonnaise, eggs, onion, scallion, garlic, almond flour, salt, and black pepper in a large bowl and mix until well combined.

Make 8 equal-sized oblong shaped patties from the mixture.

Heat the olive oil in a large skillet over medium-high heat and fry the croquettes in 2 batches for about 2-4 minutes per side.

With a slotted spoon, transfer the croquettes onto a paper towel-lined plate to drain completely.

Serve warm.

Brussels Sprout Chips

Total time: 35 minutes

Ingredients:

½ pound Brussels sprouts, thinly sliced

4 tablespoons Parmesan cheese, grated and divided

1 tablespoon olive oil

1 teaspoon garlic powder

Salt and ground black pepper, as required

Directions

Preheat the oven to 400 degrees F. Lightly grease a large baking sheet.

Place the Brussels sprout slices, 2 tablespoons of Parmesan cheese, oil, garlic powder, salt, and black pepper in a large mixing bowl and toss to coat well.

Arrange the Brussels sprout slices onto prepared baking sheet in an even layer.

Bake for about 18-20 minutes, tossing once halfway through.

Remove from oven and transfer the Brussels sprout chips onto a platter.

Sprinkle with the remaining cheese and serve.

Cauliflower Popcorns

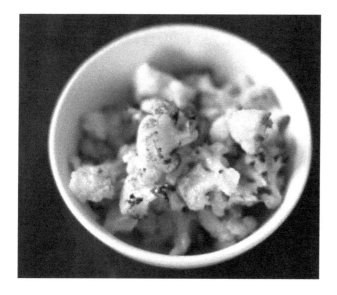

Total time: 45 minutes

Ingredients:

4 cups large cauliflower florets

2 teaspoons butter, melted

Salt, as required

3 tablespoons Parmesan cheese, shredded

Directions

Preheat the oven to 450 degrees F. Grease a roasting pan.

Add all the ingredients except Parmesan in a large bowl and toss to coat well.

Place the cauliflower florets into prepared roasting pan and spread in an even layer.

Roast for about 25-30 minutes.

Remove from oven and transfer the cauliflower popcorns onto a platter.

Sprinkle with the Parmesan cheese and serve.

Cheese Crackers

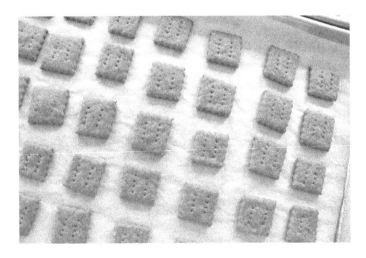

Total time: 34 minutes

Ingredients:

2 ounces cream cheese

1 cup Parmesan cheese, grated

1 cup Romano cheese, grated

1 cup almond flour

1 organic egg

1 teaspoon dried rosemary

¼ teaspoon Cajun seasoning

Salt, as required

Directions

Preheat the oven to 450 degrees F and line a baking sheet with parchment paper.

Place the cream cheese, Parmesan cheese, Romano cheese, and almond flour in a microwave-safe bowl and microwave on High for about 1 minute, stirring once halfway through.

Remove from microwave and immediately, stir the mixture until well combined.

Set aside to cool for about 2-3 minutes.

In the same bowl of cheese mixture, add the egg, rosemary, seasoning, and salt and mix until a dough forms.

Arrange the dough between 2 large parchment papers and place onto a smooth surface.

With a lightly floured rolling pin, roll the dough into a thin layer.

Remove the upper parchment paper and with a knife, cut the dough into desired-sized crackers.

Carefully, arrange the crackers onto prepared baking sheet in a single layer about 1-inch apart.

Bake for about 6-7 minutes per side or until crispy.

Remove from oven and let the crackers cool completely before serving.

Enjoy!

Cheese Bites

Total time: 20 minutes

Ingredients:

8 ounces provolone cheese, shredded

½ teaspoon paprika

Directions

Preheat the oven to 400 degrees F and line a baking sheet with parchment paper.

With a spoon, place the cheese in small heaps onto the prepared baking sheet, leaving about 1-inch apart.

Sprinkle evenly with paprika and bake for about 8-10 minutes.

Remove from oven and let the chips cool completely before serving.

Serve.

Cheese Chips

Total time: 30 minutes

Ingredients:

3 tablespoons coconut flour

½ cup strong cheddar cheese, grated and divided

¼ cup Parmesan cheese, grated

2 tablespoons butter, melted

1 organic egg

1 teaspoon fresh thyme leaves, minced

Directions

Preheat the oven to 350 degrees F and line a baking sheet with parchment paper.

Place the coconut flour, ¼ cup of grated cheddar, Parmesan, butter, and egg and mix until well combined.

Set the mixture aside for about 3-5 minutes.

Make 8 equal-sized balls from the mixture.

Arrange the balls onto prepared baking sheet in a single layer about 2-inch apart.

With your hands, press each ball into a little flat disc.

Sprinkle each disc with the remaining cheddar, followed by thyme.

Bake for about 13-15 minutes or until the edges become golden brown.

Remove from the oven and let them cool completely before serving.

Serve.

Cheddar Biscuits

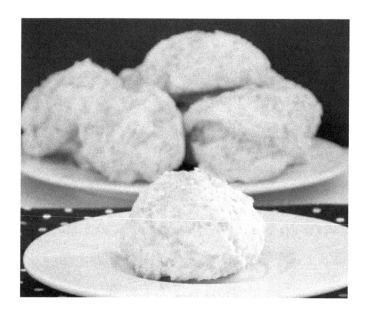

Total time: 30 minutes

Ingredients:

1/3 cup coconut flour, sifted

¼ teaspoon organic baking powder

Salt, as required

4 organic eggs

¼ cup butter, melted and cooled

1 cup cheddar cheese, shredded

Directions

Preheat the oven to 400 degrees F and line a large cookie sheet with a greased piece of foil.

In a large bowl, add the flour, baking powder, and salt and mix until well combined.

In another bowl, add the eggs and butter and beat until smooth.

Add egg mixture into the bowl of flour mixture and beat until well combined.

Fold in the cheddar cheese.

With a tablespoon, place the mixture onto prepared cookie sheet in a single layer and with your fingers, press slightly.

Bake for 15 minutes or until top becomes golden brown.

Remove the cookie sheet from oven and place onto a wire rack to cool for about 5 minutes.

Carefully, invert the biscuits onto wire rack to cool completely before serving.

Serve.

Cinnamon Cookies

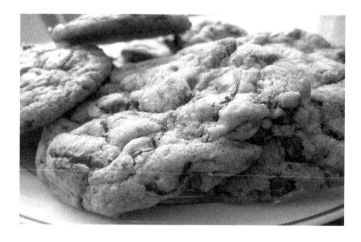

Total time: 40 minutes

Ingredients:

2 cups almond meal

1 teaspoon ground cinnamon

1 organic egg

½ cup salted butter, softened

1 teaspoon liquid stevia

1 teaspoon organic vanilla extract

Directions

Preheat the oven to 300 degrees F and grease a large cookie sheet.

Place all the ingredients in a large bowl and mix until well combined.

Make 15 equal-sized balls from the mixture.

Arrange the balls onto prepared baking sheet about 2-inch apart.

Bake for about 5 minutes.

Remove the cookies from oven and with a fork, press down each ball.

Bake or about another 18-20 minutes.

Remove from oven and place the cookie sheet onto a wire rack to cool for about 5 minutes.

Carefully, invert the cookies onto the wire rack to cool completely before serving.

Serve.

Chocolate Fat Bombs

Total time: 25 minutes

Ingredients:

8 ounces cream cheese, softened

½ cup crunchy almond butter

½ cup unsalted butter, softened

½ cup golden monk fruit sweetener

2 ounces 70% dark chocolate, finely chopped

Directions

Add the cream cheese, almond butter, butter, and monk fruit sweetener in a bowl and with an electric mixer, mix until well blended.

Transfer the mixture into refrigerator for about 30 minutes.

Remove from refrigerator and fold in the chopped chocolate.

Make 24 equal-sized balls from the mixture.

Arrange the balls onto 2 parchment-lined baking sheets in a single layer and freeze for about 45 minutes before serving.

Serve.

Mini Blueberry Bites

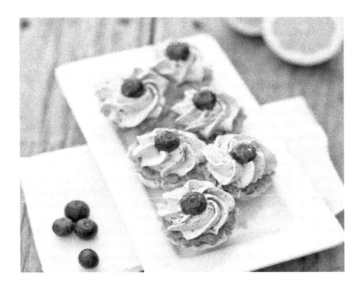

Total time: 25 minutes

Ingredients:

1 cup almond flour

½ cup pecans

½ cup fresh blueberries

4 ounces soft goat cheese

1 teaspoon organic vanilla extract

½ teaspoon stevia powder

¼ cup unsweetened coconut, shredded

Directions

Add the flour, pecans, blueberries, goat cheese, vanilla extract and stevia in a food processor and pulse until mixed completely.

Make 30 equal-sized balls from the mixture.

Coat the balls with shredded coconut.

Arrange the balls onto a parchment-lined baking sheet in a single layer and freeze for about 30-40 minutes before serving.

Serve.

Chocolate Coconut Bars

Total time: 28 minutes

Ingredients:

1 cup coconut oil

½ can full-fat coconut milk

½ cup desiccated coconut

1 tablespoon coconut flour

1 teaspoon organic vanilla extract

¼ cup cacao powder

¼ cup coconut oil, melted

4-5 drops liquid stevia

Directions

For coconut filling: add 1 cup of coconut oil and coconut milk in a pan over low heat and cook for about 2-3 minutes, stirring continuously.

Add the desiccated coconut and stir to combine

In the pan of coconut milk mixture, add the coconut flour, 1 tablespoon at a time and cook until the mixture resembles a porridge, beating continuously.

Remove the pan of mixture from heat and stir in vanilla extract.

Set the mixture aside to cool for about 10 minutes.

Place the coconut mixture evenly into a loaf pan and with the back of a spoon, press in 1-inch thick layer.

With a plastic wrap, cover the loaf pan and freeze for at least 5 hours or up to overnight.

Remove from the freezer and set aside at room temperature for about 20-25 minutes.

Place the cacao powder, melted coconut oil and stevia in a bowl and beat until well combined.

Cut the coconut filling into 9 equal-sized bars.

Dip each bar into the cacao powder mixture.

Arrange the bars onto a wax paper lined baking sheet and freeze until set before serving.

Serve.

Intermittent Fasting Salad Recipes

Salad Wraps

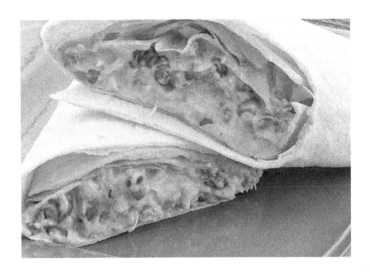

Total time: 30 minutes

Ingredients:

1 tablespoon olive oil

1 teaspoon cumin seeds

1 small yellow onion, thinly sliced

4 cups zucchini, grated

½ teaspoon red pepper flakes, crushed

Salt and ground black pepper, as required

8 large lettuce leaves, rinsed and pat dried

¼ cup Parmesan cheese, shredded

2 tablespoons fresh chives, finely minced

Directions

In a medium skillet, heat the oil over medium-high heat and sauté the cumin seeds for about 1 minute.

Add the onion and sauté for about 4-5 minutes.

Add the zucchini and cook for about 5-7 minutes or until done completely, stirring occasionally.

Stir in the red pepper flakes, salt, and black pepper and remove from the heat.

Arrange the lettuce leaves onto a smooth surface.

Divide the zucchini mixture evenly onto each lettuce leaf.

Top with the Parmesan and fresh chives and serve immediately.

Fresh Veggie Salad

Total time: 30 minutes

Ingredients:

2 cups cucumber, spiralized with blade C

1 cup Kalamata olives, pitted and halved

2 cups grape tomatoes, halved

1 tablespoon fresh oregano, chopped

1 tablespoon fresh basil, chopped

1 garlic clove, minced

2 tablespoons olive oil

2 tablespoons balsamic vinegar

Salt and ground black pepper, as required

Directions

Place all the ingredients in a large serving bowl and toss to coat well.

Serve immediately.

Berries & Spinach Salad

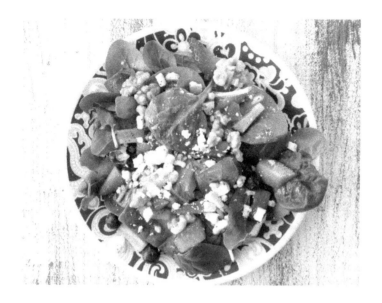

Total time: 20 minutes

Ingredients:

For Salad:

8 ounces fresh baby spinach

¾ cup fresh strawberries, hulled and sliced

¾ cup fresh blueberries

¼ cup feta cheese, crumbled

For Dressing:

1/3 cup olive oil

2 tablespoons fresh lemon juice

¼ teaspoon liquid stevia

1/8 teaspoon paprika

1/8 teaspoon garlic powder

Salt, as required

Directions

For salad: in a bowl, mix together the spinach, berries and almonds.

For dressing: in another small bowl, add all the ingredients and beat until well combined.

Place the dressing over salad and gently, toss to coat well.

Serve immediately.

Cabbage Salad

Total time: 20 minutes

Ingredients:

For Salad:

4 cups green cabbage, shredded

¼ onion, thinly sliced

1 teaspoon lime zest, grated freshly

3 tablespoons fresh cilantro, chopped

For Dressing:

¾ cup mayonnaise

2 teaspoons fresh lime juice

2 teaspoons chili sauce

½ teaspoon Erythritol

2 garlic cloves, minced

Directions

For salad: in a bowl, mix together the cabbage, onion, lime zest and cilantro.

For dressing: in another small bowl, add all the ingredients and beat until well combined.

Place the dressing over salad and gently, toss to coat well.

Cover and refrigerate to chill before serving.

Cucumber & Spinach Salad

Total time: 20 minutes

Ingredients:

For Dressing:

5 tablespoons olive oil

4 tablespoons plain Greek yogurt

2 tablespoons fresh lemon juice

2 tablespoons fresh mint leaves, finely chopped

1 teaspoon Erythritol

Salt and ground black pepper, as required

For Salad:

3 cups cucumbers, peeled, seeded and sliced

10 cups fresh baby spinach

¼ of medium yellow onion, sliced

Directions

For dressing: add all the ingredients in a bowl and beat until well combined.

Cover and refrigerate to chill for about 1 hour.

In a large serving bowl, mix together all the salad ingredients.

Place dressing over salad and toss to coat well.

Serve immediately.

Broccoli Salad

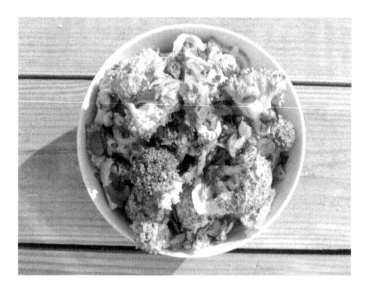

Total time: 20 minutes

Ingredients:

For Salad:

8 cups small fresh broccoli florets

1 (8-ounces) package Colby-Monterey Jack cheese, cubed

2 cups fresh strawberries, hulled and sliced

¼ cup fresh mint leaves, chopped

For Dressing:

1 cup mayonnaise

1 teaspoon balsamic vinegar

2 teaspoons Erythritol

Salt and ground black pepper, as required

Directions

For salad: in a large serving bowl, add all the ingredients and mix well.

For the dressing: in another bowl, add all the ingredients and beat until well combined.

Place the dressing over salad and gently, stir to combine.

Serve immediately.

Tomato & Mozzarella Salad

Total time: 20 minutes

Ingredients:

4 cups cherry tomatoes, halved

1½ pounds mozzarella cheese, cubed

¼ cup fresh basil leaves, chopped

¼ cup olive oil

2 tablespoons fresh lemon juice

1 teaspoon fresh oregano, minced

1 teaspoon fresh parsley, minced

2-4 drops liquid stevia

Salt and ground black pepper, as required

Directions

In a salad bowl, mix together the tomatoes, mozzarella and basil.

In another small bowl, place the remaining ingredients and beat until well combined.

Place dressing over salad and toss to coat well.

Serve immediately.

Mixed Veggie Salad

Total time: 25 minutes

Ingredients:

For Dressing:

1 small avocado, peeled, pitted and chopped

¼ cup plain Greek yogurt

1 small yellow onion, chopped

1 garlic clove, chopped

2 tablespoons fresh parsley

2 tablespoons fresh lemon juice

For Salad:

6 cups fresh spinach, shredded

2 medium zucchinis, cut into thin slices

½ cup celery, sliced

½ cup red bell pepper, seeded and thinly sliced

½ cup yellow onion, thinly sliced

½ cup cucumber, thinly sliced

½ cup cherry tomatoes, halved

¼ cup Kalamata olives, pitted

½ cup feta cheese, crumbled

Directions

For dressing: in a food processor, add all the ingredients and pulse until smooth.

For the salad: in a salad bowl, add all the ingredients and mix well.

Place the dressing over salad and gently, toss to coat well.

Serve immediately.

Creamy Shrimp Salad

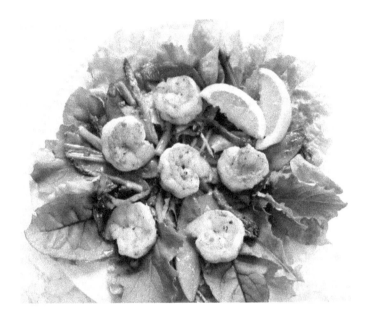

Total time: 23 minutes

Ingredients:

4 pounds large shrimp

1 lemon, quartered

3 cups celery stalks, chopped

1 yellow onion, chopped

2 cups mayonnaise

2 tablespoons fresh lemon juice

1 teaspoon Dijon mustard

Salt and ground black pepper, as required

Directions

In a pan of lightly salted boiling water, add the shrimp, and lemon and cook for about 3 minutes.

Drain the shrimps well and let them cool.

Then, peel and devein the shrimps.

In a large bowl, add the cooked shrimp and remaining ingredients and gently, stir to combine.

Serve immediately.

Intermittent Fasting Meat Recipes

Bacon Swiss Beef Steaks

Serves: 4

Prep Time: 25 mins

Ingredients

- ½ cup Swiss cheese, shredded

- 4 beef top sirloin steaks

- 6 bacon strips, cut in half

- Salt and black pepper, to taste

- 1 tablespoon butter

Directions

1. Season the beef steaks generously with salt and black pepper.

2. Put butter in the skillet and heat on medium low heat.

3. Add beef top sirloin steaks and cook for about 5 minutes per side.

4. Add bacon strips and cook for about 15 minutes.

5. Top with Swiss cheese and cook for about 5 minutes on low heat.

6. Remove from heat and dish out on a platter to serve.

Nutrition Amount per serving

Calories   385

Total Fat 25.4g   33%

Saturated Fat 10.7g   54%

Cholesterol 96mg   32%

Sodium 552mg   24%

Total Carbohydrate 0.8g   0%

Dietary Fiber 0g   0%

Total Sugars 0.2g

Protein 35.5g

Mexican Taco Casserole

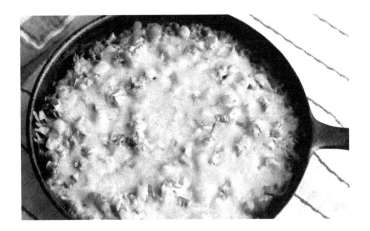

Serves: 3

Prep Time: 35 mins

Ingredients

- ½ cup cheddar cheese, shredded

- ½ cup low carb salsa

- ½ cup cottage cheese

- 1 pound ground beef

- 1 tablespoon taco seasoning

Directions

1. Preheat the oven to 425OF and lightly grease a baking dish.

2. Mix together the taco seasoning and ground beef in a bowl.

3. Stir in the cottage cheese, salsa and cheddar cheese.

4. Transfer the ground beef mixture to the baking dish and top with cheese mixture.

5. Bake for about 25 minutes and remove from the oven to serve warm.

Nutrition Amount per serving

Calories   432

Total Fat 20.4g   26%

Saturated Fat 10g   50%

Cholesterol 165mg   55%

Sodium 526mg   23%

Total Carbohydrate 3.2g   1%

Dietary Fiber 0g   0%

Total Sugars 1.6g

Protein 56.4g

Mustard Beef Steaks

Serves: 4

Prep Time: 40 mins

Ingredients

- 2 tablespoons butter

- 2 tablespoons Dijon mustard

- 4 beef steaks

- Salt and black pepper, to taste

- 1 tablespoon fresh rosemary, coarsely chopped

Directions

1. Marinate the beef steaks with Dijon mustard, fresh rosemary, salt and black pepper for about 2 hours.

2. Put the butter and marinated beef steaks in a nonstick skillet.

3. Cover the lid and cook for about 30 minutes on medium low heat.

4. Dish out when completely cooked and serve hot.

Nutrition Amount per serving

Calories   217

Total Fat 11.5g   15%

Saturated Fat 5.7g   29%

Cholesterol 91mg   30%

Sodium 186mg   8%

Total Carbohydrate 1g   0%

Dietary Fiber 0.6g   2%

Total Sugars 0.1g

Protein 26.3g

Beef Roast

Serves: 6

Prep Time: 55 mins

Ingredients

- 2 pounds beef

- Salt and black pepper, to taste

- 1 cup onion soup

- 2 teaspoons lemon juice

- 1 cups beef broth

Directions

1. Put the beef in a pressure cooker and stir in the beef broth, lemon juice, onion soup, salt and black pepper.

2. Lock the lid and cook at High Pressure for about 40 minutes.

3. Naturally release the pressure and dish out on a platter to serve.

Nutrition Amount per serving

Calories   307

Total Fat 10.2g   13%

Saturated Fat 3.7g   19%

Cholesterol 135mg   45%

Sodium 580mg   25%

Total Carbohydrate 2.9g   1%

Dietary Fiber 0.3g   1%

Total Sugars 1.3g

Protein 47.9g

Keto Minced Meat

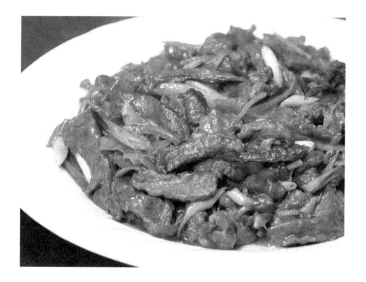

Serves: 4

Prep Time: 30 mins

Ingredients

- 1 pound ground lamb meat

- 1 cup onions, chopped

- 2 tablespoons ginger garlic paste

- 3 tablespoons butter

- Salt and cayenne pepper, to taste

Directions

1. Put the butter in a pot and add garlic, ginger and onions.

2. Sauté for about 3 minutes and add ground meat and all the spices.

3. Cover the lid and cook for about 20 minutes on medium high heat.

4. Dish out to a large serving bowl and serve hot.

Nutrition Amount per serving

Calories   459

Total Fat 35.3g   45%

Saturated Fat 14.7g   73%

Cholesterol 133mg   44%

Sodium 154mg   7%

Total Carbohydrate 4.8g   2%

Dietary Fiber 0.6g   2%

Total Sugars 1.2g

Protein 28.9g

Keto Taco Casserole

Serves: 8

Prep Time: 55 mins

Ingredients

- 2 pounds ground beef

- 1 tablespoon extra-virgin olive oil

- Taco seasoning mix, kosher salt and black pepper

- 2 cups Mexican cheese, shredded

- 6 large eggs, lightly beaten

Directions

1. Preheat the oven to 360OF and grease a 2 quart baking dish.

2. Heat oil over medium heat in a large skillet and add ground beef.

3. Season with taco seasoning mix, kosher salt and black pepper.

4. Cook for about 5 minutes on each side and dish out to let cool slightly.

5. Whisk together eggs in the beef mixture and transfer the mixture to the baking dish.

6. Top with Mexican cheese and bake for about 25 minutes until set.

7. Remove from the oven and serve warm.

Nutrition Amount per serving

Calories   382

Total Fat 21.6g   28%

Saturated Fat 9.1g   45%

Cholesterol 266mg   89%

Sodium 363mg   16%

Total Carbohydrate 1.7g   1%

Dietary Fiber 0g   0%

Total Sugars 0.4g

Protein 45.3g

Keto Burger Fat Bombs

Serves: 10

Prep Time: 30 mins

Ingredients

- ½ teaspoon garlic powder

- 1 pound ground beef

- Kosher salt and black pepper, to taste

- ¼ (8 oz.) block cheddar cheese, cut into 20 pieces

- 2 tablespoons cold butter, cut into 20 pieces

Directions

1. Preheat the oven to 375OF and grease mini muffin tins with cooking spray.

2. Season the beef with garlic powder, kosher salt and black pepper in a medium bowl.

3. Press about 1 tablespoon of beef into each muffin tin, covering the bottom completely.

4. Layer with small piece of butter and add 1 more tablespoon of beef.

5. Top with a piece of cheese in each cup and press the remaining beef.

6. Transfer to the oven and bake for about 20 minutes.

7. Allow to slightly cool and dish out to serve hot.

Nutrition Amount per serving

Calories   128

Total Fat 7g   9%

Saturated Fat 3.7g   19%

Cholesterol 53mg   18%

Sodium 81mg   4%

Total Carbohydrate 0.2g   0%

Dietary Fiber 0g   0%

Total Sugars 0.1g

Protein 15.2g

Ice-Burgers

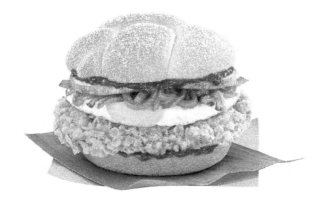

Serves: 4

Prep Time: 30 mins

Ingredients

- 4 slices bacon, cooked and crisped

- 1 large head iceberg lettuce, sliced into 8 rounds

- 1 pound ground beef

- 4 slices cheddar cheese

- Kosher salt and black pepper, to taste

Directions

1. Make 4 large patties out of ground beef and season both sides with salt and black pepper.

2. Grill for about 10 minutes per side and top with cheddar cheese slices.

3. Place one iceberg round on a plate and layer with grilled beef.

4. Place a slice of bacon and close with second iceberg round.

5. Repeat with the remaining ingredients and serve warm.

Nutrition Amount per serving

Calories   452

Total Fat 24.6g   32%

Saturated Fat 11.2g   56%

Cholesterol 152mg   51%

Sodium 698mg   30%

Total Carbohydrate 6.3g   2%

Dietary Fiber 1.2g   4%

Total Sugars 2g

Protein 49.3g

Jamaican Jerk Pork Roast

Serves: 3

Prep Time: 35 mins

Ingredients

- 1 tablespoon butter

- 1/8 cup beef broth

- 1 pound pork shoulder

- 1/8 cup Jamaican jerk spice blend

- Salt, to taste

Directions

1. Season the pork with Jamaican jerk spice blend.

2. Heat the butter in the pot and add seasoned pork.

3. Cook for about 5 minutes and add beef broth.

4. Cover with lid and cook for about 20 minutes on low heat.

5. Dish out on a serving platter and serve hot.

Nutrition Amount per serving

Calories   477

Total Fat 36.2g   46%

Saturated Fat 14.3g   72%

Cholesterol 146mg   49%

Sodium 212mg   9%

Total Carbohydrate 0g   0%

Dietary Fiber 0g   0%

Total Sugars 0g

Protein 35.4g

Pork Carnitas

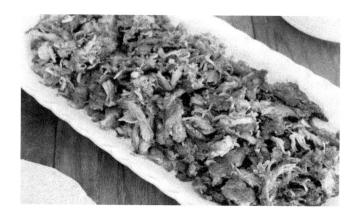

Serves: 3

Prep Time: 40 mins

Ingredients

- 1 pound pork shoulder, bone-in

- Salt and black pepper, to taste

- 1 tablespoon butter

- 1 orange, juiced

- ½ teaspoon garlic powder

Directions

1. Season the pork with salt and black pepper.

2. Put butter in the pressure cooker and add garlic powder.

3. Sauté for 1 minute and add seasoned pork.

4. Sauté for 3 minutes and pour orange juice.

5. Lock the lid and cook on high pressure for about 20 minutes.

6. Naturally release the pressure and dish out.

7. Shred the pork with a fork and transfer back to the cooker.

8. Sauté for about 3 minutes and serve warm.

Nutrition Amount per serving

Calories   506

Total Fat 36.3g   46%

Saturated Fat 14.3g   72%

Cholesterol 146mg   49%

Sodium 130mg   6%

Total Carbohydrate 7.6g   3%

Dietary Fiber 1.5g   5%

Total Sugars 5.8g

Protein 35.9g

Intermittent Fasting Fish & Seafood Recipes

Garlic Butter Salmon

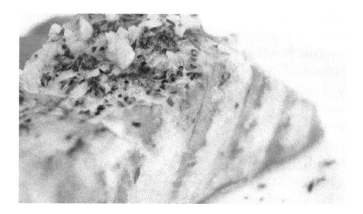

Serves: 8

Prep Time: 40 mins

Ingredients

- Kosher salt and black pepper, to taste

- 1 pound (3 pounds) salmon fillet, skin removed

- 4 tablespoons butter, melted

- 2 garlic cloves, minced

- ¼ cup parmesan cheese, freshly grated

Directions

1. Preheat the oven to 350 0F and lightly grease a large baking sheet.

2. Season the salmon with salt and black pepper and transfer to the baking sheet.

3. Mix together butter, garlic and parmesan cheese in a small bowl.

4. Marinate salmon in this mixture for about 1 hour.

5. Transfer to the oven and bake for about 25 minutes.

6. Additionally, broil for about 2 minutes until top becomes lightly golden.

7. Dish out onto a platter and serve hot.

Nutrition Amount per serving

Calories   172

Total Fat 12.3g   16%

Saturated Fat 6.2g   31%

Cholesterol 50mg   17%

Sodium 196mg   9%

Total Carbohydrate 0.8g   0%

Dietary Fiber 0g   0%

Total Sugars 0g

Protein 15.6g

Tuscan Butter Salmon

Serves: 4

Prep Time: 35 mins

Ingredients

- 4 (6 oz) salmon fillets, patted dry with paper towels

- 3 tablespoons butter

- ¾ cup heavy cream

- Kosher salt and black pepper

- 2 cups baby spinach

Directions

1. Season the salmon with salt and black pepper.

2. Heat 1½ tablespoons butter over medium high heat in a large skillet and add salmon skin side up.

3. Cook for about 10 minutes on both sides until deeply golden and dish out onto a plate.

4. Heat the rest of the butter in the skillet and add spinach.

5. Cook for about 5 minutes and stir in the heavy cream.

6. Reduce heat to low and simmer for about 3 minutes.

7. Return the salmon to the skillet and mix well with the sauce.

8. Allow to simmer for about 3 minutes until salmon is cooked through.

9. Dish out and serve hot.

Nutrition Amount per serving

Calories   382

Total Fat 27.5g   35%

Saturated Fat 12.2g   61%

Cholesterol 129mg   43%

Sodium 157mg   7%

Total Carbohydrate 1.2g   0%

Dietary Fiber 0.3g   1%

Total Sugars 0.1g

Protein 34g

Mahi Mahi Stew

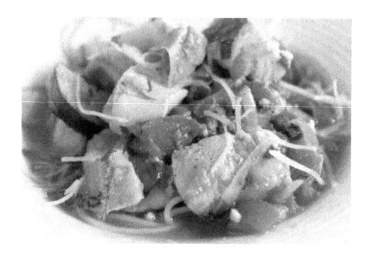

Serves: 3

Prep Time: 45 mins

Ingredients

- 2 tablespoons butter

- 2 pounds Mahi Mahi fillets, cubed

- 1 onion, chopped

- Salt and black pepper, to taste

- 2 cups homemade fish broth

Directions

1. Season the Mahi Mahi fillets with salt and black pepper.

2. Heat butter in a pressure cooker and add onion.

3. Sauté for about 3 minutes and stir in the seasoned Mahi Mahi fillets and fish broth.

4. Lock the lid and cook on High Pressure for about 30 minutes.

5. Naturally release the pressure and dish out to serve hot.

Nutrition Amount per serving

Calories   398

Total Fat 12.5g   16%

Saturated Fat 6.4g   32%

Cholesterol 290mg   97%

Sodium 803mg   35%

Total Carbohydrate 5.5g   2%

Dietary Fiber 1.5g   5%

Total Sugars 2.2g

Protein 62.3g

Sour Cream Tilapia

Serves: 3

Prep Time: 3 hours 10 mins

Ingredients

- ¾ cup homemade chicken broth

- 1 pound tilapia fillets

- 1 cup sour cream

- Salt and black pepper, to taste

- 1 teaspoon cayenne pepper

Directions

1. Put tilapia fillets in the slow cooker along with rest of the ingredients.

2. Cover the lid and cook on low for about 3 hours.

3. Dish out and serve hot.

Nutrition Amount per serving

Calories   300

Total Fat 17.9g   23%

Saturated Fat 10.7g   54%

Cholesterol 107mg   36%

Sodium 285mg   12%

Total Carbohydrate 3.9g   1%

Dietary Fiber 0.2g   1%

Total Sugars 0.4g

Protein 31.8g

Tilapia with Herbed Butter

Serves: 6

Prep Time: 35 mins

Ingredients

- 2 pounds tilapia fillets

- 12 garlic cloves, chopped finely

- 6 green broccoli, chopped

- 2 cups herbed butter

- Salt and black pepper, to taste

Directions

1. Season the tilapia fillets with salt and black pepper.

2. Put the seasoned tilapia along with all other ingredients in an Instant Pot and mix well.

3. Cover the lid and cook on High Pressure for about 25 minutes.

4. Dish out in a platter and serve hot.

Nutrition Amount per serving

Calories   281

Total Fat 10.4g   13%

Saturated Fat 4.3g   21%

Cholesterol 109mg   36%

Sodium 178mg   8%

Total Carbohydrate 9g   3%

Dietary Fiber 2.5g   9%

Total Sugars 1.9g

Protein 38.7g

Roasted Trout

Serves: 4

Prep Time: 45 mins

Ingredients

- ½ cup fresh lemon juice

- 1 pound trout fish fillets

- 4 tablespoons butter

- Salt and black pepper, to taste

- 1 teaspoon dried rosemary, crushed

Directions

1. Put ½ pound trout fillets in a dish and sprinkle with lemon juice and dried rosemary.

2. Season with salt and black pepper and transfer into a skillet.

3. Add butter and cook, covered on medium low heat for about 35 minutes.

4. Dish out the fillets in a platter and serve with a sauce.

Nutrition Amount per serving

Calories   349

Total Fat 28.2g   36%

Saturated Fat 11.7g   58%

Cholesterol 31mg   10%

Sodium 88mg   4%

Total Carbohydrate 1.1g   0%

Dietary Fiber 0.3g   1%

Total Sugars 0.9g

Protein 23.3g

Sour Fish with Herbed Butter

Serves: 3

Prep Time: 45 mins

Ingredients

- 2 tablespoons herbed butter

- 3 cod fillets

- 1 tablespoon vinegar

- Salt and black pepper, to taste

- ½ tablespoon lemon pepper seasoning

Directions

1. Preheat the oven to 375OF and grease a baking tray.

2. Mix together cod fillets, vinegar, lemon pepper seasoning, salt and black pepper in a bowl.

3. Marinate for about 3 hours and then arrange on the baking tray.

4. Transfer into the oven and bake for about 30 minutes.

5. Remove from the oven and serve with herbed butter.

Nutrition Amount per serving

Calories   234

Total Fat 11.8g   15%

Saturated Fat 2.4g   12%

Cholesterol 77mg   26%

Sodium 119mg   5%

Total Carbohydrate 0.4g   0%

Dietary Fiber 0g   0%

Total Sugars 0.1g

Protein 31.5g

Cod Coconut Curry

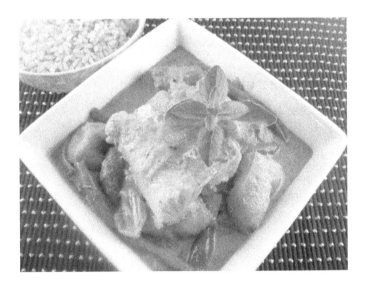

Serves: 6

Prep Time: 35 mins

Ingredients

- 1 onion, chopped

- 2 pounds cod

- 1 cup dry coconut, chopped

- Salt and black pepper, to taste

- 1 cup fresh lemon juice

Directions

1. Put the cod along with all other ingredients in a pressure cooker.

2. Add 2 cups of water and cover the lid.

3. Cook on High Pressure for about 25 minutes and naturally release the pressure.

4. Open the lid and dish out the curry to serve hot.

Nutrition Amount per serving

Calories   223

Total Fat 6.1g   8%

Saturated Fat 4.5g   23%

Cholesterol 83mg   28%

Sodium 129mg   6%

Total Carbohydrate 4.6g   2%

Dietary Fiber 1.8g   6%

Total Sugars 2.5g

Protein 35.5g

Garlic Shrimp with Goat Cheese

Serves: 4

Prep Time: 30 mins

Ingredients

- 4 tablespoons herbed butter

- Salt and black pepper, to taste

- 1 pound large raw shrimp

- 4 ounces goat cheese

- 4 garlic cloves, chopped

Directions

1. Preheat the oven to 375OF and grease a baking dish.

2. Mix together herbed butter, garlic, raw shrimp, salt and black pepper in a bowl.

3. Put the marinated shrimp on the baking dish and top with the shredded cheese.

4. Place in the oven and bake for about 25 minutes.

5. Take the shrimp out and serve hot.

Nutrition Amount per serving

Calories   294

Total Fat 15g   19%

Saturated Fat 8.9g   44%

Cholesterol 266mg   89%

Sodium 392mg   17%

Total Carbohydrate 2.1g   1%

Dietary Fiber 0.1g   0%

Total Sugars 0.8g

Protein 35.8g

Grain Free Salmon Bread

Serves: 6

Prep Time: 35 mins

Ingredients

- ½ cup olive oil

- ¼ teaspoon baking soda

- ½ cup coconut milk

- 2 pounds salmon, steamed and shredded

- 2 pastured eggs

Directions

1. Preheat the oven to 375ºF and grease a baking dish with olive oil.

2. Mix together coconut milk, eggs, baking soda and salmon in a bowl.

3. Pour the batter of salmon bread in the baking dish and transfer into the oven.

4. Bake for about 20 minutes and remove from the oven to serve hot.

Nutrition Amount per serving

Calories   413

Total Fat 32.4g   42%

Saturated Fat 8.5g   42%

Cholesterol 138mg   46%

Sodium 143mg   6%

Total Carbohydrate 1.5g   1%

Dietary Fiber 0.4g   2%

Total Sugars 0.7g

Protein 31.8g

Best Exercises to Lose Weight

With these myths in mind, let's move on to some science about the combination of fasting and exercise or 'fasted workouts'. These workouts are very popular for morning fasts since you can wake up with a relatively empty stomach, have some water, and hit your workout. However, there is much controversy on the subject of exercise on an empty stomach. There are not many studies available on the practice specifically, so the debate continues. Whether or not you think it works better than exercise on a half-full stomach or not, this book is here to give you suitable information to make your own informed decisions.

So, we know that when the stomach is empty, and the body has no immediate access to energy, then it will rely on stored fats. This fact alone implies that working out during a fast would successfully burn unneeded fat reserves, thus leading to weight loss. Although weight loss is the main focus here, we also need to address the many other benefits that IF has when combined with exercise. Studies have shown that fasted cycling to enhance endurance was easier to recover from than endurance cycling with food in the stomach. Along with recovery from endurance exercises, we have seen an improved recovery from the wear and tear of weight training, so we see a pattern of improved recovery after a workout if the athlete was in a fasted state. Similarly, fasted workouts should have higher glycogen storage. By keeping glycogen levels low during workouts, your body adapts to running on low glycogen. Thus, when you have food in your stomach, the body will use its energy more efficiently since it is trained to do so.

These ideas may not be the most amazing practices for a professional athlete, but for a regular person looking to shed a few pounds or develop a new lifestyle, the practices seem optimal.

But what about the many different types of exercise?

Most experts agree that exercise is safe to do while on an empty stomach, but are you getting the most out of your workout? As far as we can tell, the following conclusions can be found:

If your workout requires high levels of speed and power, you will benefit from having food in your stomach. This is due to the high amount of energy you will be burning in a short amount of time, so the energy that is available to be burned quickly is ideal for getting the most out of your workout.

For an empty stomach or fasted workout, the experts suggest cardio and aerobic workouts on all levels, whether it's tai chi or a jog through the park, or intensive yoga and deep stretching. These less intense workouts are ideal practices during a fast and will be the most effective for weight loss.

It is also understood that if you wish to start a fasted cardio routine, you should not have any serious health conditions like low blood pressure or other conditions that may cause dizziness or increase the risk of injury. The following tips are a great guideline for beginners:

1. Stay hydrated. Consume plenty of water.

2. Do not work out for longer than an hour

3. Choose moderate or low-intensity workouts

4. Listen to your body. If you experience discomfort, then take a breather

In the following chapters, we will reference 'light exercise'. This may be self-explanatory, but it will not hurt to suggest some exercise practices that pair well with IF. These exercises are light and not tough on the body, but we should still break a nice sweat when we are performing these 'light' exercises.

Some fitting ideas for fasted exercise:

- **Yoga**

Sanskrit for 'union', this traditional Indian practice sets out to unite the body and mind by combining intricate poses and stretches with structured breathing exercises. Cultural influence aside, even spending ten to fifteen minutes a day dedicated to stretching the body and focusing some attention on deep breathing will do wonders as a warmup to a workout or a workout in and of itself.

You can find plenty of books and online resources to find a yoga practice that suits you. The practice aims to strengthen the body while also furthering flexibility. It is a great core workout and really assists us in getting to know our body and its boundaries.

- Tai Chi

As a traditional Chinese martial art, this practice is designed to teach the practitioner how to control and manipulate the subtle energies of the body and its surroundings. Somewhat similar to yoga, this practice involves the constant movement of postures rather than holding poses. Breath is just as important during tai chi as in yoga. As a general rule, being in control of your breathing is a key component to a mindful and healthy life.

There is an abundant amount of material on tai chi online, and many major cities have multiple tai chi instructors and classes that meet in groups or one-on-one. Finding a class that takes place in a natural or relaxing setting is ideal.

- **Jogging**

All of us are familiar with jogging. The casual running exercise aims to build endurance and stamina by running at a steady pace at moderate speeds. Early morning jogs are a great way to start the day and pair well with a fasted morning.

You can jog anywhere. Jog around the block of your neighborhood or visit a school track or a gym that has running space to change the scenery. There are many running groups online if you feel uncomfortable running alone.

- **Cardio**

Cardio workouts are defined as any workout that gets your heart rate up. Jogging can be considered cardio, but there are meticulously designed cardio workouts that aim to burn fat through different intensities. Many workouts ask that you have intervals of intense cardio followed immediately by rest than more intense cardio.

There are hundreds of different cardio styles and workouts available online to suit your skill level and lifestyle. Your local gym should have machines perfect for cardio and possibly even classes dedicated to weight loss through cardio. Cycling machines and the elliptical are popular machines you can find at gyms for cardio workouts.

- **Pilates**

Very similar to yoga, but with more strength building exercises, Pilates was invented in the twentieth century as an effective way to tone muscle without bulking up. It pairs well with IF since it is low impact and can be performed anywhere, not unlike yoga.

Most cities should have Pilates instructors nearby, and there are abundant resources online.

- **Hiking**

This is a low-impact, relaxing, and thought-provoking activity. Taking a hike in the woods is an immersive experience. There's something very beneficial about being in a natural setting away from all the hustle and bustle of a town or city. Depending on the terrain, hiking can be a casual stroll or close to a treacherous climb. The combination of fasting and hiking is an amazing one as you notice your senses are heightened as you walk empty-bellied through the forest.

There are hiking trails all around the world, and they often state the intensity level of the hike. Searching for new trails and scenic spots quickly becomes a hobby that is beneficial on many levels. Adventurous, educational, self-reflective, and most certainly great for your body, hiking is paired wonderfully with IF since you are in control of how difficult it is. But, of course, if you are fasting and going out into the woods, be sure to bring plenty of water and emergency snacks.

How to Overcome Down Moments

It really doesn't matter whether you are a newbie to intermittent fasting or you've been at it for a while. Each day you struggle to the finishing post, to the small window of time when you can eat but it seems that everywhere you look, people are eating delicious meals and sipping on full-fat flavored coffees. You find yourself resenting them while you sit and sip on a black coffee or a bottle of water, counting down the minutes and hours until you can eat again. Is that you? Most people who do on intermittent fast go through exactly the same thing but there is one way to get over it and that is to change your mindset and build up good healthy habits.

It's very easy to fall into the trap of thinking in a certain way. Many people who have tried dieting find themselves in a diet mindset – you are either on one or you aren't. You are either being good or you are cheating on your diet. And, it follows, that you are either losing weight or gaining it.

The same goes for intermittent fasting. You will, without a doubt, go at it with the same mindset – you'll reach your goal and then you'll work out how to maintain it. The biggest problem is that too many people see intermittent fasting as a temporary fix to the temporary problem of weight gain. The actual problem is in mindset. You must learn to see intermittent fasting as a permanent way of life and the only way to fix your mindset is to change it permanently. You need to shed the diet mindset and then you will start to see the results you want. You are no longer on a diet, there is no longer a point at which you stop. This is for life and the sooner you realize that, the easier it will become.

Now, this is the most important part of all. You will find yourself in another mindset – the 'can't' mindset. I can't eat until 6 pm. I can't eat when everyone else is easting. I can't add cream and sugar to my coffee. Instead of focusing on enjoying your lifestyle, you will be focusing on what you see as deprivation. Instead of thinking about what you can do, you constantly think about what you can't do.

This is the mindset you need to shake off quickly because, until you do, you can't even enjoy intermittent fasting and, believe me, it is an enjoyable lifestyle.

Instead of telling yourself that you deserve to eat when everyone else is, you need to tell yourself that you deserve your health and you deserve to lose weight more.

Make that change and you'll find yourself cooking for your family without even thinking about whether you can eat or not.

How do you conquer the 'can't' mindset? How easy is it? Some people will find it easier than others but the one thing you should do is read and re-read the benefits of doing intermittent fasting. Weight loss may be your goal, but intermittent fasting is about so much more. It's about cleansing your body and slowing the aging process. It's about improving your health and having more energy. It's about rediscovering yourself, the person that you are meant to be.

You need to understand that it has nothing to do with not being able to eat when you want; it's all about choosing not to. It's about choosing to understand that your body doesn't need that much food. It's about understanding that your body will benefit from you eating the right foods but giving your body a chance to recuperate and recover every day. It's about watching the fat melt away with just one simple change to your life. Where's the hardship in that? Where's the deprivation when you find yourself fitting into clothes you never thought you'd ever be able to wear again?

The only thing you are "depriving" yourself of is bad health.

So, are you ready to make a huge change in your life? Change your mindset and you'll be happier and healthier than you ever knew. And this all leads to something else – a change in your eating habits.

Because you can only eat during a certain window of time, you'll want to make the most of it. By feeding your body healthy nutritious and delicious foods, you won't want to go back to eating junk. Sure, you can 'treat' yourself occasionally, but I promise you this – after a while on intermittent fasting, once your body gets used to eating a healthier diet, you won't want those treats.

One more thing you need to understand – this won't happen overnight. You have to work at changing both your mindset and your habits so be patient and give yourself time.

F.A.Q. About Intermittent Fasting

Is an Intermittent Fasting Diet the Right Choice For Me?

So does an intermittent fasting diet work when compared to other diets? The answer here is a resounding yes. For example, using a 16 hour fast will keep your body burning fat for most of every day! And getting all of your calories during a relatively small eating window stops your body from going into starvation mode and desperately hanging onto body-fat. Compared to a normal reduced calorie diet, this is a huge difference. While any reduced calorie approach will initially lead to fat-loss, your body is an efficient machine and will compensate by slowing down your metabolism (the exact opposite of what you want) and holding onto body fat.

Is an intermittent fasting diet restrictive? Any diet, by its very nature, involves making better food choices. If someone tries to sell you on the pancake diet, run a mile! Eating rubbish can never be a good choice. However, most diets will have you try to eat clean all the time. This is very hard to do and is directly linked to finding yourself eating 12 doughnuts in one sitting after a couple of weeks of deprivation! Intermittent fasting also involves healthy food choices, but it does give you more wiggle room. It is difficult to eat to much junk in a small eating window after you have already had your healthy food. It does let you eat enough to stop you falling off the wagon, however.

Perhaps the real advantage of intermittent fasting is that it can be a lifestyle rather than a short-term approach. With most diets, even if you do manage to follow it long enough to get results tend to be followed by a rebound- that is a return to poor eating and fat gain. By viewing fasting as a long-term solution, this problem effectively disappears.

Should I take vitamins when I intermittently fast?

It is more important than ever to take vitamins and supplements when fasting, as you are skipping meals that were helping to supply you with these vital nutrients and it's important that you replace them. The biggest problem with vitamins and fasting is that taking a vitamin pill in a fasted state may result in stomach pain, nausea, and diarrhea. To avoid these unpleasant, unsettling effects, try and get your vitamins down while in the fed state. If this is impossible, try taking your vitamins at night so you can sleep through the discomfort.

Alternatively, you might choose vitamins in liquid form, as they are easier to digest while fasting. If you don't normally take vitamins, a basic multivitamin that provides 100% of your daily intake is a great start to ensure you aren't missing out on anything while intermittently fasting.

Why would anyone fast who doesn't want to lose weight?

It may seem odd to someone who is considering intermittently fasting to lose weight, for anyone who has their weight under control to change their eating habits or patterns. After all, aren't they already living the dream? Let's not forget about all the other benefits of intermittent fasting:

• Fasting for health benefits: Some people swear by fasting because they feel it improves their sleep, mental clarity, and helps them control and maintain chronic diseases such as diabetes, cardiovascular disease, multiple sclerosis, fibromyalgia, chronic fatigue syndrome, cancer and the side effects from chemotherapy.

• Fasting for athletes: Fasting offers a consistent method of fueling and resting the body that works under many of the same principles as training and rest days. It offers them a much more convenient way to ensure that they consume the food they need to train than the other option of eating small meals every 2 or 3 hours, and it allows them to maintain a nutrition routine that provides a lengthier feeding time which can be enjoyed with friends and family.

- Fasting for busy people with poor eating habits: People who travel a lot for business often end up feeling less than well most of the time, due to poor eating habits developed as a result of airport restaurants and late-night vending machines.

- Make sure you are well-hydrated and avoid salty or sugary foods before you fast.

- Don't stuff yourself the night before you fast. This "last supper" mentality is a rookie mistake that will give you indigestion, a poor night's sleep, and an even ruder awakening to your stomach and brain when you follow up the preceding evening's bacchanalia with a fasting period.

Why do I get headaches when I fast and how can I stop them?

Complaints of headaches especially when beginning an intermittent fasting program are quite common. If you are waking with a headache, you may not have hydrated yourself enough the night before. Not drinking enough water is one of the biggest culprits of headaches during fasting and water should be imbibed throughout the fasting/feeding process. Headaches can also be a side effect of the detoxing process that occurs in intermittent fasting and will be especially prevalent in the beginning stages of incorporating the program into your health regime.

Isn't intermittent fasting just a fancy way of saying I'm starving myself?

• Fatty acids are used by the body as an energy source for muscles but lower the amount of glucose that travels to the brain. Fatty acids also include a chemical called glycerol that can be used, like glucose as an energy source, but it too will eventually run out.

• Fat stores are depleted, and the body turns to stored protein for energy, breaking down muscle tissue. The muscle tissue breaks down very quickly. When all sources of protein are gone, cells can no longer function.

• The body does not have the energy to fight off bacteria and viruses. It takes 8 to 12 weeks to starve to death, although there have been cases of people surviving 25 weeks or more.

Is intermittent fasting safe for women?

Women are more hormonally sensitive than men. Because of this, they may respond more intensely to the challenges of intermittent fasting and need to consult with a medical professional before starting an intermittent fasting program, especially if they have menstrual and fertility issues. Once intermittent fasting has been undertaken, women should also pay special attention to their menstrual cycle, and seek medical guidance if they begin missing periods.

There is a modified technique of intermittent fasting that will help women who experience hormonal sensitivity. This is a more progressive approach that will help the female body adapt to fasting.

- Fast for 12-16 hours

- On fasting days, stick to light workouts such as yoga or light cardio

- Fast on 2-3 nonconsecutive days per week

- After a few weeks, add another day of fasting and monitor how it goes.

- Drink loads of water

- Save strength training for feeding periods or feeding days

Why can't I have a protein shake when I'm fasting?

You can't eat food when you are intermittently fasting – hence you can't drink a protein shake. People get confused about protein shakes – check out diet, fitness, and nutrition and health websites if you don't believe me. I used to shake my head in wonder when I first saw this question asked.

If you are on a 5:2 type of intermittent fasting program and you are consuming 500 to 600 calories on your "low" days, feel free to indulge in one or 2 of these shakes if they don't bring you over your total calorie count. If you are on Whole Day Fasting or in the fasting portion of your Time Restricted intermittent fasting cycle, don't even think about it!

How can I fast when I'm on vacation?

I indirectly referred to the answer to this question when I was explaining some of the advantages of Whole Day Fasting and 5:2 Intermittent Fasting. Because you are confining your fasting to 2 non-consecutive days of the week, you can automatically end up with a 4-day feeding unit of time. This will help the eating challenges of holidays and vacations in a big way.

Conclusion

Surely, intermittent fasting has so much to offer without compromising one's appetite or health. The advantage IF offers over other diet plans is that you do not need to restrict yourself to eating something that you do not like.

Intermittent fasting does not give you a dieting schedule to follow. Rather, it focuses on a fasting routine that will let your body recover after working hard to digest your food every day. All these biological functions give you a better body that has lost a considerable amount of fat. Intermittent fasting has several benefits that you cannot deny.

It gives you the opportunity to stay fit and healthy without losing your ability to enjoy your food to the fullest. However, that does not mean you should exploit this routine by cheating during your eating hours. Even if you are not on a diet or fasting plan, you should not add junk food to your diet. That will simply deplete your energy and keep killing you from the inside.

As you learned, IF has many benefits to offer. While several of them lack proper backing by research, it is certain that intermittent fasting does help with weight loss. As you know, some of the deadliest conditions, like diabetes, are linked to obesity. With a controlled weight, you will eliminate such illnesses.

The result is a win-win situation in which you do not have to compromise your health. Just remember to practice intermittent fasting in moderation in the beginning so that you get used to it. Once you feel comfortable with your schedule, you can increase the number of hours you fast so that you can work on your health with even more dedication.

Furthermore, combining intermittent fasting with a capable diet plan like the Keto diet will give you more benefits. It will help you switch to fat (instead of carbs) as the main source of energy for your body. That way, your body will become balanced and healthy. Achieving that level is tough, but with practice, you can reach it and enjoy a much healthier lifestyle.

Hopefully, you have enjoyed reading this book. Look for healthy recipes that will suit your lifestyle and give you the comfort you need every day.

CPSIA information can be obtained
at www.ICGtesting.com
Printed in the USA
BVHW080953120521
607048BV00009B/2637